Superfood Smoothies

The 101 Best Super Smoothie Recipes for Healthy Living and Weight Loss

By

Michelle Brighton

Table of Contents

Introduction

By now I hope that you have read at least one of my books in my superfood series and know a bit more about me but, in case you haven't, let me go through things for you.

Today, I am healthy, vital, and full of energy and no longer look my age – I look a lot younger. I am at the pinnacle of health and no longer even have a scale in my house.

This was not always the case. In fact, if you had seen me as I am today and me as I was 10 years ago, you would be forgiven for thinking we were two different people.

You see, the *me* back then was, quite frankly, completely lost. I was fat, kept gaining weight and was sick and tired all time. I had given up on trying to lose weight and resigned myself to the misery that my life had become.

I had given up on ever being thin and healthy again and, quite frankly, nothing in my life at the time was such an issue that I felt forced to make a real change. I wasn't happy about the way that I looked and I knew it was not healthy for me, but I couldn't motivate myself to care.

Basically, it wasn't until I hit rock bottom that I started to make lasting changes in my life. It all started with a pain in my arm – and no, this is not a story about a heart attack – the pain initially wasn't so bad, more of a nuisance really. Then it moved up into my shoulder and all the way down the left side of my body.

And then it got worse. In fact, I was in such agony that the doctor ordered x-rays, thinking that I had injured my vertebrae. All that the x-rays picked up, fortunately, was that my muscles were in spasm.

I was give pain relievers and the pain subsided and so life went back to normal again.

Okay, now you are wondering where the life changing part of this came in – for the next few years, I played cat and mouse with the pain – I'd have an attack, get medication and then be alright for a while again.

Then the medication stopped working and the attacks began to get more frequent and severe. I went back to the doctor and was told it was a pinched nerve, and that I would have to take medication for the rest of my life. A second and third doctor disagreed about the cause of the pain but also prescribed a life-time course of medication.

It was there that I decided enough was enough. I was not going to destroy my body even more by taking strong painkillers every day and so I decided to do my own research.

I learned about superfoods and about changing your life slowly, one step at a time and the results were astonishing. I adopted one healthy new food a week and did a little exercise and started to feel better, without medication.

And now, I feel great and I want you to feel great as well. Start by swapping out your breakfast for a smoothie every day and I guarantee that you will see great results, just as I did.

Want it made easy for you? In this book we cover both the basics that are needed when making a smoothie so that you can design your own and 101 different, super-healthy smoothie recipes for those days when you need a little inspiration.

Good luck!

Chapter 1:
The Benefits of Smoothies

Why incorporate smoothies in your diet at all? Let's go through it quickly.

Making Smoothies is a Quick Shortcut to Getting a Nutritious Meal, Without Worrying about Burning the Food

How long does a traditional breakfast of pancakes, eggs and sausage take to cook? Probably a lot longer than anyone in today's modern culture really has to be able to do it on a daily basis. You have to make the pancake batter, heat the skillet, fry the eggs, fry the sausages - let's say it takes a half an hour – at least.

How long for a delicious tasting, meal replacement, protein and nutrient packed smoothie? Throw the washed veggies and fruit into your blender, along with protein powder, honey, yogurt, soy milk and whatever you feel like putting in there and you have breakfast in under five minutes. Plus, you have made the very healthy decision to skip the greasy, fat-filled, high cholesterol conventional breakfast that will keep you operating as if you're in a fog for the next few hours. Smoothies are quick, tasty and just as filling as "real" meals, without making you uncomfortably full.

Smoothies Can Help Your Body Heal

If you have ever been ill for any length of time, you know how hard it becomes to sling down a full meal at mealtimes. Even when you have just gotten ill, the last thing that you usually feel like doing is to eat.

Smoothies can help you to heal your body by providing the nutrients that you need in a format that is easy to use, swallow and digest.

You can boost the healing power of the smoothie based on the condition you are suffering from – got colds or flu? Add in some ginger, honey and a little garlic and skip the dairy milk.

Just feeling wiped because of a particularly rough day at work? Restore your energy with some spirulina or wheatgrass in your smoothie.

Have an upset stomach? Peppermint or fennel in your smoothie can help restore the balance.

Smoothies give you Loads of Energy

We all are grateful when we get an extra spurt of energy. Coffee and other caffeinated drinks, along with sugary snacks give us these bursts, but they just don't last very long and the come down is difficult and always at the wrong time.

Smoothies, on the other hand, can give us a steady flow of natural energy that lasts for hours. Fruit and vegetables do that because of the amount of fiber that they contain. And when the fruits and veggies are broken down to their most absorbable size, as in a smoothie, then you're getting all the energy and nutrients that were meant for you. Smoothies provide healthful and reliable energy for athletes, students, homemakers, business people and everyone who simply needs more stamina.

Smoothies Dramatically Increase Your Fiber Intake

I am willing to bet that you are not getting enough fiber in your diet and that is a pretty safe bet considering the fiber stats for the average American. Your average American will take in about 15g of fiber daily, according to the U.S. National Library of Medicine. Sounds good, doesn't it? Until you consider that the optimum fiber intake per adult is between 25g and 38g a day.

By incorporating more smoothies into your diet, you naturally increase the amount of fiber that you consume. Fiber can help to keep your digestion working properly, help you lose weight, reduce the risk of heart disease and colon cancer, and also lower the risk of developing diabetes and/ or a stroke. Making smoothies on a daily basis will increase the intake of fiber to your diet and will help you to flush toxins from your body as well as give you a feeling of fullness, which means that you will naturally want to eat less and lose weight.

Smoothies Provide Antioxidants that Prevent Cell Damage and Help Prevent Premature Aging

Antioxidants are basically stable chemicals in the body that bind themselves to unstable chemicals known as free radicals. If left unchecked, the free radicals can wreak havoc in our body and cause a range of problems from simple inflammation to lifestyle diseases such as diabetes through to even more sinister diseases such as cancer.

The smoothie recipes in this book contain a lot in the way of fruits and vegetables, which are high in antioxidants and can help in the fight against free radicals. There are plenty of them and just a few of them are: blueberries, blackberries, strawberries, apples, kale, carrots and beets.

Smoothies can Speed Weight Loss

A smoothie a day melts the pounds away. That is the simple fact. When you replace a meal with a healthy smoothie, you can't help but to lose weight. You're getting a healthy meal in a glass instead of a long sit-down meal full of sugar, salt and some refined, indigestible, who knows what, that will take a day or more to digest. The meal replacement smoothie gives you what your body needs and gives it to you in a delicious and easily digestible manner that will help you lose the pounds fast.

Smoothies are the Easy Way to Incorporate Superfoods into Your Diet

Superfoods are special foods in a category all by themselves. They are extremely high in nutrients and generally low in calories, which can improve people's mental and physical health. Many superfoods are incorporated into my smoothie recipes. Some of them include, blueberries, kale, beets, sweet potatoes, Swiss chard, spinach, chia seeds and flax seeds, to name a few.

So if superfoods are so great, why don't we eat more of them? Put quite simply, some superfoods, like blueberries and sweet potatoes do taste great and are probably part of your diet already. Others, like kale and Swiss chard, on the other hand, are something of an acquired taste – I know that before I started taking healthy eating seriously I would buy a bunch and dump it into the fridge to prepare "later".

The kale would reproach me every time I opened the fridge until, eventually, and with a sigh of relief, I would realize that it was "past its best" and ready for the compost heap.

Smoothies make it possible to blend the not so nice ingredients with ones that taste much better. At the end of the day, you are unlikely even to taste the ones you don't like. I no longer have the salad drawer of the doomed. (Too bad for the compost heap.)

Smoothies make it simple to get a lot of superfoods into our bodies all at once in a quick, delicious way.

Chapter 2:
Smoothie Basics

If you are not a fan of the taste of kale or some other vegetable as it is, mixing it into a smoothie is a great option because you can disguise the flavor. There are a ton of smoothie recipes further along in this book but let us go into the basics of making your own smoothies so that you can mix and match as required.

With these basics in mind, you can either blend your own smoothies from scratch or switch out ingredients in any of the smoothie recipes listed in this book – the choice is yours.

Your Smoothie Liquid

Choose a base for your smoothie – this will be the liquid part of the smoothie that makes it easier to blend all the other ingredients. I like using almond milk but you can use regular milk, soy milk, fruit juice (not ideal because of all the sugar), an herbal tea or even just plain water. When I am just making the two of us, I add about half a cup of the base and water it down further with half a cup of ice – also makes for a wonderfully icy drink.

Experiment with using coconut water, herbal tea, green tea or whatever combination takes your fancy.

The more liquid you add, the runnier your smoothie will be. If, in fact, you find that the smoothie is too thick, adding a bit more liquid is the way to go.

I always add a little liquid into the base of the blender before I add my veggies and fruit – it helps things whizz together more easily.

Start with about a cup of liquid and half a cup of ice. (Omit the ice if using frozen fruit.)

Add in a Healthy Vegetable

Now, this part is not essential but you may as well add in a vegetable such as kale, carrots, etc. Any vegetable that can be eaten raw. You need not even peel it, scrub well, top and tail, cut into chunks and toss it in. The reason that we add the vegetable is to get an extra boost of fiber and nutrients and the best part is that you won't even taste it!

Add in one or two pieces of raw vegetables.

Add in Your Flavorings

Now we add the flavor and by this I mean some sort of fruit. I usually add in two different fruits for a bit of flair. Bananas and pineapples are my favorite because they are really sweet and can hide a lot of veggie flavor but add whatever fruit you fancy.

Now, I realize that the banana is high in sugar but it adds a delicious creaminess to the blend. Also, if I don't want to water down the flavor of the smoothie, I freeze my fruit and add the frozen fruit in the place of ice. (You may then need to add a little more of your base liquid is you do this)

Add in 2 small servings of fruit.

Add in Your Protein

Protein is what is going to give you lasting energy throughout the day and leave you feeling fuller for longer. Now, before you go chucking a piece of raw steak into the smoothie, there are a lot of options when it comes to protein.

To really give it a protein boost I about five almonds or cashews. If I have Chia seeds in the house, I will put about a tablespoon in just enough water to cover them and leave them overnight. By morning, they will have become gelatinous and make a great addition to the smoothie.

The milk, Chia seeds and nuts do add a good serving of protein but I will usually just add a tablespoon of whey powder to up the protein content as well.

With the protein, it depends on what you are adding but generally a tablespoonful is a good rule for whey powder and Chia seeds and about 5-10 nuts is a good quantity when it comes to nuts.

Making it More Filling

Adding in some raw oats or plain oat bran is a great way to increase the fiber content even more and to make it that much more satisfying as a meal.

Consider Spicing it Up

As for flavoring, a teaspoon of turmeric makes for a wonderful juxtaposition of flavors and can also help to boost the anti-inflammatory effects of the mixture.

Chapter 3:
Some Troubleshooting Tips

You can always add a little more liquid if your smoothie turns out too thick for your liking – alternatively, you can always eat it with a spoon.

If your smoothie is too watery, add a bit more oatmeal or a little more whey powder to thicken it up. You can also add more veggies for the same reason.

It is best to roughly chop the fruit and veggies before putting them into the blender – as an example, you could quarter an apple. This does not take long but it does make things easier on the blender and can help to extend the useful life of the blender.

Add a bit of liquid and then add the fruit and vegetables. Pulse until it is smooth and then add everything else. Leave the ice until last.

The one downside of using vegetables such as kale and spinach in a smoothie is that you are bound to get what looks like pond scum forming on top – there is nothing wrong with this foam but if you don't want to drink it, just scoop it off.

You will want to invest in a decent quality blender, especially if you plan to add in ice. If your budget does not stretch quite that far, you can use a cheaper quality blender but will need to make sure only to use the more tender parts of the fruits and vegetables, to chop them finer and to leave out the ice and frozen fruit.

Chapter 4:
Making Your Own Base Ingredients

DIY Nut Butter

Okay, so technically this is not a smoothie but I snuck this in here because it is so easy to do. This is best done in a high-power blender or a food processor.

Take a cup of nuts, a teaspoon of coconut oil, a pinch of salt and a teaspoon of honey (optional) and process until smooth.

Refrigerate and use within a week. (Mine never makes it to a week old, it always gets eaten!)

DIY Coconut Milk

Make Your Own Coconut Water

Take one green coconut and place it on an even, sturdy surface. Using your sharpest, heaviest non-serrated knife, cut through the coconut, about 2 or 3 inches from the top, as you would a jack-o'-lantern. Tip: Cutting a square opening instead of a circle will make it easier for you to extract the juice.

Check the color of the coconut flesh. It should be white. If it is pink or tan or greyish or any other color, it may be going bad.

Using a spoon, scrape away any flesh that could be in the way of the opening.

Take a peek at the coconut water (also known as coconut juice; the terms are used interchangeably). It should be clear or slightly milky with no sour smell or taste. If it is an off- color or tastes sour, the coconut water has gone bad.

Add a straw and serve in the coconut or decant into a glass. If you are not drinking it immediately, add a dash of lemon or lime juice and refrigerate. Use with two days. Alternatively, put any leftovers into ice cube trays and freeze.

Don't waste the rest of the coconut – crack it open all the way and then use the gelatinous flesh as well.

Make Your Own Coconut Milk

You will need the flesh of one mature coconut and some water. This means cracking open the coconut and scooping out as much flesh as possible. You want to make sure that you remove all of the brown rind so that only the white flesh remains.

Put the flesh to one side as we will only be working with a little at a time.

Put some of the flesh into a blender and add just enough water to cover it. Process on the highest power setting until the coconut meat is liquefied, and then pour it into a container.

Working in small batches, continue processing the coconut meat until all of it has been liquefied.

If you like, pour the blended coconut milk through a fine sieve or cheesecloth to remove any solids. (You can use the solids in baked goods, curries, and smoothies.)

Store the coconut milk in an airtight container for up to 5 days in the fridge. You can freeze any unused milk in an airtight container for up to 3 months.

Make Your Own Coconut Milk with Dried Coconut

You will need equal parts of boiling water and desiccated coconut, (unsweetened is best.)

Pour the water and coconut into your blender. Pulse on high until completely liquid.

Place in a covered container and leave undisturbed until it has cooled completely, or preferably overnight.

Strain the liquid and retain the solid matter for use in cooking.

Place the coconut milk in an airtight container. It will keep for around 5 days in the refrigerator (if you don't drink it first) and can be frozen for around 3 months.

If you want to make a different quantity, the rule is simple – equal parts water and coconut.

DIY Almond Milk

Making almond milk is really simple – I soak a cup of almonds overnight in water and then discard the water in the morning. Place the almonds in your blender and add 3 cups of water and a teaspoon of vanilla extract. Pulse until smooth, decant and refrigerate. Use within 2-3 days. I like the grit at the bottom and usually leave it in when making my smoothies but if it is a problem for you, you can strain it out. Don't throw it out though – it makes a really great skin scrub. Alternatively, mix it in with your muesli or porridge or eat it as it is.

Using Raw Sprouts

When it comes to promoting healthy digestion, there is little better that you can do than to eat raw food as far as possible. Raw food contains some digestive enzymes that can help promote good digestion.

These enzymes, however, can be destroyed by cooking so, where you can, it is best to eat raw foods. In addition, cooking will also break down some of the fiber in the food and this, again, is not good for promoting a healthy digestive system.

Raw food can help to feed the healthy bacteria in the gut and so restore balance.

Prebiotics can help to feed the healthy bacteria in the gut without overdosing your system. Prebiotics are basically foods that are high in fiber and more difficult for the body to digest. Because of this, these substances pass through the stomach and are processed in the gut.

Prebiotics that can be of use include lentils, beans and chickpeas.

Chickpeas can be enjoyed in a number of different ways and are a very versatile snack food. Roast some chickpeas in the oven with a drizzle of olive oil and seasoning to taste for a healthy alternative to crisps. Alternatively, you can cook the chickpeas and incorporate them into you morning smoothie or make them into hummus.

The easiest way to incorporate these foods into your diet when raw is to grow your own sprouts. Sprouts are easy and quick to grow – all you need is a bottle and some muslin to cover the opening of the jar.

Cover the seeds in water and soak for about half an hour. Strain off the water and leave the sprouts in a cool, dark place. Repeat every morning and evening until the seeds start to sprout – depending on the seed this can be in as little as 3 -5 days. Mung beans and alfalfa will grow in two or three days, chickpeas can take a week.

Whilst not strictly necessary, I did find that a seed sprouter was a good investment to make and I do advise you to consider getting one yourself if you find that you enjoy sprouting vegetables.

The sprouter has a series of trays that are perforated to make it easy for water to drain off the sprouts. You simply place your sprouts on the trays and pour water over the top layer. The water filters down through all the layers and the excess collects in the tray for this purpose. The trays make things more convenient because they nestle on top of one another neatly and they allow you to more easily separate out your different sprouts. I have five trays going at any one time to ensure a steady supply of sprouts and enough variety.

When the seeds have grown about a centimeter, they are ready to eat or be thrown into your smoothie. Eat at least a handful at a time – they provide amazing amounts of energy and are amongst the most nutritious foods on the planet. The leftovers can stay in the bottle or tray and will grow as long as you keep watering them. For best benefits though, eat within a couple of days of sprouting.

It is important to use food quality seeds for sprouting and not seeds intended for planting. Seeds that are intended for planting have usually been treated with poisons to help them stay healthy.

How to Make the Recipes in This Book

You will notice that I have only provided the recipes in this book and not the instructions as well. That is because the procedure is basically always the same, no matter what recipe you are making and I did not want to bore you by repeating it over and over again.

It is simple – get all the ingredients together. Try to minimize preparation by only peeling fruit and vegetables where absolutely necessary – I don't even core my apples. Basically, as long as the blender can handle it, put it into the blender. Chop roughly – I usually make thumb length pieces at smallest.

On that note, blenders do not do well with hard stones such as peach pits and date pits so do remove these before adding to the blender.

Start by putting a little of the base liquid into the blender. Then add the toughest of the materials you are blending – this will usually be your pumpkin seeds, if you are using them, and vegetables. Pulse until smooth and then add in your fruits and the rest of your liquid. Add the ice, if you are using it, last of all.

Now there is bound to be some sort of residue that is left at the bottom of the blender that does not get completely incorporated – I usually spoon this out and eat it.

Smoothie to Go

Streamlining the process makes it even easier, especially if you are really pressed for time in the morning. Prepare whatever you can ahead of time – what I do is to portion out the nuts and seeds that I will be using for the week ahead and store them in little containers. I do the same with the fruit and freeze it ahead of time.

I usually prep the veggies the night before – this is best done closer to the time for optimal freshness.

Then it is a simple matter of grabbing the nut and seed mix, my bag of fruit, the milk/ water and my veggie. Smoothies done in half the time on a busy, rushed morning.

Measuring out your ingredients ahead of time can also help with portion control – it can be quite easy to forget how many nuts we should add or to underestimate or overestimate the size of a portion.

One note here – I did once think that it would be time saving to make double or triple batches of the smoothies in order to save time later. They never look or taste as good the following day and I suspect that they also lose a lot of nutrients as well.

Only make enough to drink in one day – I will often make a batch that is enough for my morning lunchtime meal. I don't push it any farther though. Besides, they really are so easy to make, you don't need to.

Chapter 5:
Kale Smoothies

I personally know that kale does not make it onto most people's lists when it comes to their favorite foods but it is one of the most nutrient dense of all foods on the planet. It definitely deserves a place in everyone's diet. In fact, if you choose to incorporate only one recipe from this book at all, make sure that it comes from this section.

If the flavor is a problem for you, smoothies are definitely the answer. Smoothies are an easy way to sneak in healthy foods so that you really do not taste them and they taste fantastic.

Need More Convincing?

Kale has more Vitamin C in it than the same amount of orange would have. It is a little known fact that kale is one of the richest sources of Vitamin C on the planet and the nutrients don't stop there.

In fact, one cup of raw kale contains:

206% of your daily requirement of Vitamin A

684% of your daily requirement of Vitamin K

134% of your daily requirement of Vitamin C

9% of your daily requirement of Vitamin B6

26% of your daily requirement of Manganese

9% of your daily requirement of Calcium

10% of your daily requirement of Copper

9% of your daily requirement of Potassium

6% of Magnesium

In addition, it also contains some Vitamin B1, Vitamin B2, Vitamin B3, Vitamin E, Phosphorous and Iron.

Vitamin A

Vitamin A in the form of beta carotene is one of the primary nutrients found in kale. Vitamin A doesn't get as much press as the B Vitamins or Vitamin C but it is every bit as important.

Studies have shown that it is a strong anti-inflammatory in its own right and that it is a very important in helping to ward off premature aging, being especially useful in preventing wrinkles and hyperpigmentation associated with aging.

It is also important for the respiratory tract – helping to kill off respiratory tract infections and being especially useful in getting rid of pneumonia. It is also helpful in reducing the symptoms of asthma.

Not enough for you? It can rid the body of fungal infections such as candida, help fight bacterial infections and also viral infections it an all-round important booster for the immune system and in the fight against disease.

It helps to improve fertility and will help to prevent a low birth weight in babies.

It is great for the eyes, helping to increase photosensitivity (hence the common conception that it will help you see in the dark) and helps to halt the progression of macular degeneration.

Vitamin B1 (Thiamin)

The vitamin works wonders in maintaining nervous system and muscle health, as well as helping the body convert sugar to usable energy.

Brown rice, seeds, and legumes (such as lentils and beans) are terrific sources of vitamin B1. Kale does not contain as much vitamin B1 as these sources, but it is a good, easy way to add thiamin to your daily diet.

VITAMIN B2 (Riboflavin)

This special nutrient plays several roles, including helping the body to maintain its supply of other B-complex vitamins, protecting the cells from free-radical damage and supporting cellular energy production. It also helps to prevent and treat anemia, carpal tunnel syndrome, cataracts, dry eyes, eye conditions including sensitivity to light and blurry vision, recurring headaches (including migraines), rosacea, and skin rashes.

Kale is a good source of this important vitamin. I've got to be completely honest: kale does not contain the extreme riboflavin levels that cremini mushrooms, spinach and venison do, but it is an easy way to get more of this essential B-complex vitamin into your diet.

Vitamin B3 (Niacin)

Like its 8-complex cousins, niacin helps the body with energy production at a cellular level. It is also necessary to sustain healthy levels of cholesterol, stabilize blood sugar, help the body process fats, and help the cells create new DNA. That's a lot of important jobs for one nutrient! Don't get enough vitamin 83 and you may feel tired and lethargic-you may even experience muscle weakness, digestive upset, or skin rashes.

Kale contains moderate amounts of most 8 complex vitamins, including vitamin 83. One cup of cooked kale contains .65 mg of niacin, which is 3.2 percent of an adult 50 daily recommended allowance. Every little bit counts!

VITAMIN B6

Vitamin B6 was initially identified as a skin healing vitamin but we have learned that it has a much greater role in the body. It will help to reduce inflammation and treat inflammatory skin conditions such as allergic reactions, eczema and psoriasis but will also help with treating cardiovascular disease, depression, nerve problems related to diabetes and carpal tunnel syndrome.

It has been shown valuable in managing the symptoms of epilepsy and autism as well as alleviate the effects of alcoholism, adrenal gland dysfunction, asthma, HIV/AIDS, kidney stones, PMS, and vaginitis, Vitamin B6 has also been used to reduce pregnancy-related nausea, prevent the loss of brain function in Alzheimer's patients, lower the risk of lung cancer, and even to help break up kidney stones, With all that, it's no wonder that vitamin B6 is the most thoroughly studied of the B-complex vitamins.

Vitamin B9 (Folate or Folic Acid)

If you have been trying to fall pregnant, you will no doubt have heard of folic acid. Folic acid can help to ward off birth defects, particularly those of the neural tube. It can also help to protect your growing baby from disorders of the nervous system.

It is just as useful for adults though – it can stave off the onset of dementia and Alzheimer's disease, can lower the risk of developing cancers of the lung and esophagus, intestine, cervix and uterus. It can also reduce your risk of developing osteoporosis and keeps the skin healthy.

Vitamin C (Ascorbic Acid)

Vitamin C was the first-discovered-and remains one of the best known of the antioxidant vitamins, meaning it fights oxidation in the body. You probably already know what oxidation is: Think of a cut apple. What happens when its flesh is exposed to air: It gets brown, right? That's oxidation. A small bit of oxidation happens naturally in the body during regular cell function.

BUI unsafe levels of oxidation can occur when you are exposed to steady amounts of pollution, chemicals, processed food, excess sugar, alcohol, cigarette smoke, and even stress. The result is cell damage and even death. Oxidation makes our skin look older, our immunity weaker, and our bodies more prone to fatigue and illness.

Vitamin C can help the body ward off oxidation by a complex chemical reaction that kills oxidized cells. It also helps with wound healing, maintains healthy tissue (from skin tissue to gum tissue to the tissue that makes up our blood vessels), and boosts the immune system.

Fortunately, kale is packed with this hardworking nutrient. One cup of kale provides 134% of your daily requirement of Vitamin C.

Vitamin E (Tocopherol)

This is one of nature's most potent antioxidants and it is actually not just one molecule but rather a group of molecules that are similar in structure and that work together synergistically.

These molecules help to mop up free radicals and work at boosting your immune system, protecting your nervous system and bolstering the cardiovascular system.

1 cup of kale gives you about 5.6% of the daily recommended allowance which, admittedly, does not seem like a whole lot but it is not bad for such a hard-working little vegetable.

Vitamin K

Vitamin K has been pretty much ignored until recently because we didn't really understand how important it was in the prevention of osteoporosis and helping with strengthening the skeletal system.

In addition, it helps to prevent excessive bruising and bleeding and helps with ensuring that the blood clots properly.

Kale is arguably the best food source of Vitamin K.

Carotenoids

Carotenoids are what Mother Nature uses to color in with. In other words – the beet gets it red color from carotenoids just as the carrot does. There are hundreds of different carotenoids that scientists have been able to isolate, but this might just only be the tip of the iceberg.

These include beta-carotene, alpha-carotene, gamma-carotene, lycopene, lutein, betacryptoxanthin, zeaxanthin, and astaxanthin. Carotenoids happen to be powerful anti-oxidants that protect and strengthen human cells-each carotenoid provides slightly different benefits, but overall, they work to increase immune system function and fight off the damages of free radicals in the body.

If you are not eating a range of different fruit and vegetables a day, you are not getting enough carotenoids in your diet. You could, for example, just be eating kale and still not be getting enough – variety is just as important here.

Being deficient in carotenoids leaves you open to lowered fertility, reduced immune function, increased risk of lifestyle and dread diseases and open to premature aging.

Long-term low intake of carotenoids-which is not uncommon among people who don't eat several servings of veggies a day-can make you susceptible to infertility, lowered immunity against infectious diseases, and an increased risk of cardiovascular diseases and cancers. It can also diminish the quality of your skin, hair, and nails.

Whilst there is no official daily minimum requirement for carotenoids, it is generally agreed that one should be eating a minimum of 5 fruits and veggies a day for maximum benefits.

Flavonoids

Flavonoids are also pigments found in nature but only those found in plants. They are also great antioxidants. There have be thousands identified already and, again, scientists believe that this is only the tip of the ice berg.

Flavonoids fulfil a similar function in the body to carotenoids when it comes to preventing the cells of the body from degenerating. In research conducted in Europe, it was discovered that those with the highest intake of flavonoids reduced their risk of stroke by a whopping 20%.

Again, there are no official recommended daily allowances for flavonoids but if you have your 5 servings of veggies a day you will be fine. Kale has a lot of these health-giving compounds.

Glucosinolates

These are phytonutrients that contain sulfur compounds that are especially useful when it comes to lowering the risk of developing cancer and also helping cancer patients to overcome their cancer.

These compounds are also essential when it comes to beating inflammation and are one of the building blocks that NAC (see below) needs to make glutathione. These compounds can help rid the body of toxic residue and put an end to inflammatory conditions.

Again, no daily recommended amount has been laid out but you can be sure of getting the glucosinolates that you need by having three servings of kale a week.

Fiber

Fiber gives structure to food. In plant food, such as kale, it provides the tell-tale shape of the leaf (or stalk, root, tuber, bulb, flower, pod, or seed). Fiber is essential if you hope to have a healthy digestive system.

Basically there are two types of fiber – soluble and insoluble. Soluble fiber is digested and helps to slow the rate at which glucose is released into the blood stream, thereby regulating blood sugar levels. In addition, fiber is harder for the body to digest than say a molecule of sugar would be and this further slows things down when it comes to your blood sugar levels.

Insoluble fiber is not digested and basically sits in your tummy, making you feel fuller until it is moved into the intestinal system. Once there, it helps to make it easier for the body to process the waste materials by bulking them out.

Insoluble fiber is also an essential food source for those friendly bacteria in the gut, and keeps their populations healthy, further facilitating the complete digestion of your food.

If you want to get the best possible value out of your food and truly want to be in great health, fiber is essential. The problem with the traditional Western diet is that it is generally too low in fiber and too high in processed foods.

Fiber is essential to good health. A cup of kale provides about 10% of the fiber that you need for the day.

Omega-3 Fatty Acids

I am sure that you will know something in regards to Omega-3 fatty acids. These healthy fats help to fight inflammation and are essential for the good health of our hair, nails and skin.

A deficiency of these oils will leave you less able to focus and more likely to be depressed and irritable.

Omega-3s boost your immunity and have been found to help reduce dangerous abdominal fat as well.

The anti-inflammatory properties of these fats make them essential in reducing the risk of cardiovascular disease, cancer, stroke, IBS and rheumatoid arthritis.

And the body is unable to produce its own Omega-3s so it is essential to get them from food. A cup of kale will give you about 5.4% of the recommended daily allowance of Omega-3.

Protein

Whether you are an adherent of the low-carb diets like Banting and keto or not, there is probably no doubt that you understand how important protein is in our diets. Protein is essential for most body functions – from the very building of the cells to regulating the body's fluid balance.

Those who are pregnant, or who have been injured or are recovering from illness, those who are endurance athletes and those who do very physical work and children need more protein than normal.

This is one area were the Western diet is not so bad – we do tend to get enough protein.

Protein is an essential part of the diet because it provides a great deal of energy and it packs a punch in terms of keeping you feeling full for longer.

Kale has about 4.9% of protein per cup so it is not bad in that respect.

Calcium

The "Got Milk" campaign drummed into us exactly how important calcium is to us but, with the current backlash against dairy products, many of us are not getting sufficient calcium anymore and this is a worry – without enough calcium in your diet, your bones will become more brittle and breaks and fractures will take longer to heal.

But that is not all – you can also expect to experience aching muscles, muscles that spasm and even pins and needles.

If a child does not get enough calcium, it can affect their growth rate and cause skeletal deformations.

What you may not realize is that kale is a pretty good source of calcium in its own right and that the calcium in it is easy for us to digest, making it a real contender when it comes to getting enough calcium.

Copper

If you were to do an analysis of trace minerals present right now in your body, you would find that copper would be one of the most common minerals. It is necessary to regulate the function of enzymes within the bodies, to help the body process and use iron, to protect against free radicals, in the creation of connective tissue and bone and also necessary to produce melanin – the skin and hair pigment.

Deficiencies are rare because there are a lot of dietary sources of copper but you can expect to have higher bad LDL cholesterol, sores on the skin, anemia, an increased propensity to developing infections, a lack of energy, aching joints, a shortness of breath, osteoporosis, a propensity towards ruptured blood vessels, problems with your heartbeat and repressed thyroid function.

Iron

Iron is another one of the nutrients that the whole body needs. Whilst iron supplementation is seldom necessary, it is possible for you to become deficient in it.

Iron molecules serve as the basis for haemoglobin in the red blood cells and these have the important function of transporting oxygen throughout the entire system.

Without iron, you would not be able to make use of the energy your body produces or metabolize the fat in the system and your immune system would be a lot weaker.

Now pundits will tell you that iron from meat sources is a lot better for you and this is actually true – the body can more easily absorb the iron in meat. That does not mean, however, that it cannot utilize the ion content of kale, it just means that it will not be able to use a lot of it.

Manganese

Manganese is not one of those nutrients that we need a lot of but a deficiency can have far-reaching effects because it is a nutrient that activates the enzymes in the body.

Deficiency can manifest as diabetes and unregulated sugar levels, skin conditions, loss of bone density, cholesterol levels that are too low (yes, that is a real thing), allergies, dizziness, asthma, loss of hearing, learning disabilities, multiple sclerosis, PMS, schizophrenia, rheumatoid arthritis, reduced fertility, vomiting, nausea, weakness of the muscles, convulsions, vertigo, paralysis, blindness and recurring sprains.

Now for the good news, by just having one cup of kale, you are getting 26% of the recommended daily allowance.

Magnesium

Back to the blood analysis of trace elements – coming second on the list of the most common minerals is magnesium. Magnesium is found in abundant quantities in the body and a lot of it is stored in the skeletal system. It is required by each and every cell in your body.

It is required for more than 300 essential biochemical reactions. It is necessary for the metabolization of fat, glucose and proteins, the creation of RNA and DNA, the production of enzymes, the production of glutathione and a stable production of cholesterol.

Your body must get enough magnesium through the diet or you risk losing it from the bones and weakening your skeletal structure.

If you have a magnesium deficiency, you can expect to experience fatigue, headaches, insomnia, muscle cramps, muscle weakness, sugar levels that are out of balance, high blood pressure, problems with your heart rate, soft, weak bones.

Phosphorus

Another mineral that is found in each cell, the highest concentration of phosphorus is, however, in the teeth and bones. This makes sense because it is the mineral most necessary for building strong teeth and bone.

It works in conjunction with the B Vitamins to aid the conduction of neural impulses and muscles contractions. It also helps to keep your heartbeat regular and improves kidney function.

It is found in a lot of food sources so a deficiency is rare so it is not that much of a big deal that kale contains moderate amounts of it.

There is an interesting fact to note here in relation to phosphorus in the soda that we drink. In America, we drink about four times as much soda as people in Europe do. Now, not only is that a bad thing because of the sugar content of the soda but also because of the phosphorus content.

If you drink a lot of soda, you may actually be getting more of this mineral that is good for you. Too much phosphorus can cause osteoporosis, loss of bone density and heart disease.

How much is too much? More than three servings a WEEK! I know people who have three lots of soda in a day.

Tryptophan

Tryptophan is no doubt an amino acid that you have hear of before – it is one that helps the body to make protein. More importantly though, it is the precursor for serotonin, the nutrient that helps you to remain calm and that can make you sleepy.

Kale contains enough tryptophan to allow you to remain calm but not so much that you feel sleepy as well after eating it.

Tryptophan will also help reduce the severity of headaches, PMT and will help to curb cravings thereby helping you to stick to a healthier eating plan.

Kale Smoothie Recipes

Apple and Kale Smoothies

(Serves 2)

2 apples

1 cup kale

1 cup coconut water

2 tablespoons honey

½ teaspoon cinnamon

½ cup oats

Triple A Smoothie

(Serves 1)

1 apple

2 apricots, pitted

½ Avocado

½ cup kale

½ cup plain yoghurt

2 tablespoons honey

½ cup water

10 ice cubes

Kale and Cucumber Smoothie

(Serves 1)

1 cucumber

1 cup kale

1 cup almond milk

½ cup freshly picked mint leaves

Juice from one lemon

10 ice cubes

Kale and Hearty Smoothie

(Serves 1)

1 cup kale

½ cup wheatgrass

1 banana

½ cup plain yoghurt

½ cup oat bran

1 tablespoons Chia Seeds that have been soaked in a little water overnight

½ cup water

10 ice cubes

Strawberry Kale Surprise

(Serves 1)

1 cup of baby kale

1 cup of strawberries

1 banana

1 cup milk of your choice

1 tablespoon of honey

8 ice cubes

Glutathione Booster

(Serves 1)

1 cup kale

½ cup cauliflower

1 clove garlic, peeled and minced

1 teaspoon of fresh ginger, peeled and finely chopped

1 cup wheat grass

1 cup of water

1 teaspoon turmeric

Antioxidant and Energy Booster

(Serves 1)

1 cup kale

1 cup of blueberries

1/2 cup of green tea

½ cup of Red Bush tea (Substitute with green tea if you cannot find it)

1 tablespoon of honey

Ice to taste

Super Green Smoothie

(Serves 1)

1 cup kale

1 cup of blueberries

1/2 cup of green tea

½ cup of Red Bush tea (Substitute with green tea if you cannot find it)

1 tablespoon of honey

Ice to taste

Kale Dessert Smoothie

(Serves 2)

If you are in need of some fast comfort food, this is your go-to shake. Please note that due to the addition of the ice-cream, it is not the healthiest of the smoothies so it should be reserved for an occasional treat.

2 cups coconut milk

1 cup chocolate chip ice cream (full fat with dark chocolate is better if you can find it)

1 cup baby kale leaves

¼ of an avocado

2 drop peppermint extract (optional)

Choco-Kale Smoothie

(Serves 2)

2 cups milk of your choice

1 cup baby kale leaves

¼ cup nut butter or a handful of nuts

1 banana

30ml of unsweetened cocoa powder

Blissful Berry

(Serves 1)

1 cup coconut water

1 cup assorted frozen berries

1 cup baby kale leaves

For the Little Ones

(Serves 2 kids)

This can be enjoyed by kids of any age – if you are making it for yourself this is enough for one adult serving. What I like about this is that it is rich and creamy and that you hardly taste the kale.

Because of the smooth texture and mild flavor, you can easily sneak the kale past your kids. (I tell mine that I put green juice in to make a cool color, they don't even realize they are eating veggies.)

1 cup milk of your choice (coconut works well in this blend)

1 cup baby kale

1/3 cup raw nuts of your choice

¼ avocado

½ banana/ pear

A teaspoon of vanilla essence

Seriously Cool Slushy

(Serves 4)

This is awesome on a hot summer's day. It has a fair amount of sugar in it so it should also be kept as an occasional treat. What I sometimes do is to freeze this mixture to make lollipops for the kiddies.

250ml baby kale leaves

½ cup homemade, unsweetened applesauce or pear sauce

500ml water or coconut water

250ml organic lemonade

About 8 ice cubes

Kale with a Kick

(Serves 2)

500ml milk of your choice

250ml baby kale leaves

¼ cup nut butter or a handful of nuts

1 banana

30ml of unsweetened cocoa powder

Kale Delight

(Serves 2)

1 banana

1 cup kale leaves (or collard greens or bok choy)

¼ cup pitted dates 1 cup arugula

1 cup milk (soy or almond milk is ok)

Kale for President

(Serves 2)

1 carrots (cleaned and chopped)

2 cups kale (leaves only, no stems)

2 ½ cups coconut water

1 ½ apples (green preferably)

¼ cup lemon juice

Tropical Dreams

(Serves 1)

2 cups pineapple chunks

1 ½ cup mango chunks

2 cups coconut water

1 ½ cups kale (chopped)

2 tablespoons chia seeds (soaked for about an hour in just enough water to cover them)

Bone-Boosting Smoothie

(Serves 2)

½ avocado

½ cup broccoli

4 tablespoon wheat bran

10 almonds

1 cup kale or spinach

1 ½ cups spring water or almond milk

Green Goodness Smoothie

(Serves 2)

4 kale leaves (chopped)

½ cup spinach (chopped)

2 ½ cups coconut water

½ cup parsley leaves (no stems)

½ cup cilantro

2 apples (green preferably)

½ ginger root (grated)

2 tablespoons blue-green algae powder

Immune Booster

(Serves 2)

½ avocado, ½ cucumber

½ pear, ¼ lemon

¼ cup cilantro

¾ inch ginger (sliced)

1 ½ cup kale (tightly packed)

¾ cup coconut water

¼ cup protein powder

2 cups water

Love Your Heart Smoothie

(Serves 2)

1 cup cucumber (peeled and sliced)

1 cup kale or spinach

1 celery stalk (chopped)

½ cup parsley (chopped)

1 tablespoon psyllium husks (or Metamucil)

1 apple (peeled and de-seeded)

2 tablespoon lemon juice

1 tablespoon lime juice

Chapter 6:
Coconut Smoothies

Now this is one health food that most people can get their heads around – coconut tastes great and provides a lot of healthy fats, fiber and energy. Whether you want to incorporate it by cooking with coconut oil or coconut milk or add it to your smoothies in the form of coconut water, milk, oil or flesh, it is up to you.

There is one caveat here – you can, if you like, use desiccated coconut on one condition – that it is unsweetened.

Why is Coconut a Health Food?

In this chapter, let us go through an overview of the benefits of coconut and a little more about the humble coconut itself.

Coconut Conquers Sweet Cravings

Natural, unsweetened coconut improves the production of insulin and facilitates the more efficient use of blood glucose. The fat in the coconut itself helps to slow down the absorption of glucose into the blood stream and so reduces spikes in sugar and subsequent crashes.

Coconut Sugar or Nectar

Both of these, as long as they are unsweetened, provide a pleasant sweet flavor and are low on the glycemic index. What this means for you is that you can eat these foods without worrying about getting a sugar rush or fueling cravings for refined carbohydrates.

Coconut and Immunity

Eating coconut on a regular basis can help to boost immune system function. Coconut oil and milk in particular have a strong anti-bacterial, anti-fungal and anti-viral action. In addition coconut is also rich in antioxidants.

Coconut and Your Skin

Because of the high levels of anti-oxidants in coconuts, they help fight the signs of aging and protect you against damage from U.V. radiation but that is not all – the fatty acids in the fruit itself can help to firm up the connective tissue in the skin - whether eaten or used directly on the skin, coconut will help you to look younger.

Coconut and Your Metabolism

The fatty acids are not just good for your skin though – they can also boost your metabolism and support the functioning of your thyroid. They will also help to support the function of the adrenal glands as well. This is particularly important if you are subjected to a great deal of stress.

Coconut Water and Electrolytic Balance

Coconut water contains electrolytes that can help balance hydration levels during exercise without all the chemicals and additives that are found in your typical sports drink.

Coconut and Satiety

In addition to being low on the glycemic index, coconut flesh also has a lot of fiber in it and this can help to contribute to feelings of satiety – you can eat less and still feel full.

Coconut and Cardiovascular Disease

Now we come up against the traditional wisdom that states that coconuts are high in fat and so bad for the cardiovascular system. In 2003 this old chestnut was finally laid to bed – scientists in Quebec at the McGill University actually found that those in the study consuming coconut oil actually had lower levels of cholesterol than those who ate red meat.

Coconuts and Weight Control

According to similar studies, in both animals and humans, the fatty acids in coconut are structured in such a way as to make one feel full faster and have a more balancing effect on the subject's weight than the more complex fatty acids that are found in meat sources.

Coconut and Real Food

Whether you have adopted the raw food, real food, gluten-free or Paleo eating plans, you will find that coconut features highly. Coconut is a "real" food with all the goodness that nature intended. It can be eaten raw with minimal preparation and that is what the new real food movement is all about.

Coconut Smoothie Recipes

Fruity Shake Up

(Serves 2)

¼ cup chopped pistachios, almonds, or skinless hazelnuts

1 cup diced ripe papaya or mango

1 small carrot, peeled and chopped

⅔ Cup freshly squeezed orange juice

1 cup coconut milk (homemade or from can, aseptic box, or refrigerated carton)

15ml lime juice

10ml coconut sugar

3 or 4 ice cubes

Nutty and Nice

(Serves 2)

1 cup coconut water

1 cup coconut milk (homemade or from can, aseptic box, or refrigerated carton)

½ cup pecan pieces

1 tablespoon chia seeds

1 banana or small, ripe peeled pear

1 teaspoon coconut nectar

1teaspoon pure vanilla extract

Pinch of sea salt

Dreamboat Smoothie

(Serves 2)

1 orange

1 cup unsweetened coconut milk (homemade or from can, aseptic box, or refrigerated carton)

1 teaspoon vanilla extract

1 tablespoon coconut oil

3 to 4 ice cubes

Tropical Zing Smoothie

(Serves 2)

1 cup fresh or frozen pineapple chunks

½ cup freshly squeezed orange juice

2 tablespoons raw pepitas (green, hulled pumpkin seeds)

1 slice ginger, peeled

1 teaspoon coconut sugar

1 tablespoon fresh lime juice

1 cup coconut milk (homemade or from can, aseptic box, or refrigerated carton)

3 or 4 ice cubes

The Ultimate Smoothie

(Serves 2)

½ avocado

½ cup coconut milk (homemade or from can, aseptic box, or refrigerated carton)

½ cup coconut water

¼ cup plain coconut yogurt or kefir

½ fresh or frozen banana

2 tablespoons coconut butter or dried unsweetened coconut

2 ice cubes

Optional: ½ teaspoon vanilla extract

Vitally Delicious and Nutritious Smoothie

(Serves 2)

1 cup coconut water

½ cup packed young coconut pulp (or ¼ cup unsweetened shredded dried coconut)

1/3 cup macadamia nuts

½ teaspoon pure vanilla extract

½ tablespoon coconut nectar

When you need a Boost Smoothie

(Serves 2)

1 cup coconut milk (homemade or from can, aseptic box, or refrigerated carton)

¼ teaspoon grated lime rind

Juice from 1 lime or two key limes

1 tablespoon coconut nectar or sugar

1 tablespoon coconut oil

¼ cup unsweetened shredded dried coconut

3 ice cubes

Place first 6 ingredients in a blender; process until smooth. Add ice cubes and pulse until smooth.

Get Your Day off on the Right Foot Smoothie

(Serves 2)

1 large handful roughly chopped kale, spinach, or collards, or a combination of these greens

1 cup frozen mango chunks

1 cup coconut water

2 tablespoons almond butter

1 tablespoon chia seeds

Optional: squirt of lemon or lime

Love Your Skin Smoothie

(Serves 2)

2 ½ cups coconut water

1 ½ oranges (sliced, peeled and seeds removed)

2 kiwis (peeled and sliced)

2 tablespoons flaxseeds (preferably ground or in powder form)

Coco-Berry Surprise with a Hint of Mint

(Serves 2)

1 ½ cups coconut water

1 ½ cups blueberries

1 ½ cups strawberries

2 teaspoon chia seeds (soaked overnight in just enough water to cover them)

¼ cup leaves of mint

2 tablespoons lemon juice

I Love Mango Smoothie

(Serves 2)

1 ½ cups pineapple chunks

1 cup mango chunks

2 ½ cups coconut water

2 tablespoons chia seeds

Anti-Stress Booster Smoothie

(Serves 2)

¾ cup dried oatmeal

¾ cup raw almonds (chopped finely)

1 ½ bananas

2 ½ cups coconut water.

2 -3 tablespoons sweetener (your choice, though honey is preferred)

Fiber Boosting Smoothie

(Serves 2)

2 cups almond milk or soymilk

½ avocado

1 pear (sliced)

1 ½ cups spinach (tightly packed)

½ cup coconut water

1 tablespoon chia seeds

½ cup protein powder

2 ½ cups water

Silky Smooth Skin Smoothie

(Serves 2)

1 apple (peeled, cored and seeds removed)

1 ½ limes (peeled, sliced and seeds removed)

¾ cup parsley (leaves only, no stems)

2 tablespoons of coconut oil

2 tablespoons of fresh mint, chopped finely

1 large cucumber (peeled)

1 cup coconut water

2 cups purified water or almond oil

MUFA Rich Smoothie

(Serves 2)

½ avocado (ripe) or 4 tablespoon almond butter

½ cucumber

1 cup kale or Bok Choy or romaine lettuce

½ banana

¾ cup blueberries

1 cup spring water or coconut water

Creamy, Chocolatey Smoothie

(Serves 2)

¼ cup cocoa powder or chocolate syrup

½ cup coconut milk 6 dates (pitted)

2 cups low fat milk or soymilk

2 tablespoon sweetener (your choice)

6 ice cubes

Coconut and Almond Smoothie

(Serves 2)

1 ½ cups coconut water 1 ½ cups almond milk

2 tablespoons honey or sweetener of your choice

1 cup cubed pineapple (fresh or frozen)

¼ cup shredded coconut

½ teaspoon vanilla extract

Minty Fresh Smoothie

(Serves 2)

1 ½ cups low fat milk or almond milk

½ cup coconut water

½ cup chocolate protein powder

2 cups frozen spinach (or 3 cups fresh spinach)

½ cup dry oats

¼ teaspoon peppermint extract

Get Your Vitamin C Smoothie

(Serves 2)

½ banana

¼ cup coconut water

¼ cup strawberries (frozen or fresh)

6 ounces plain or vanilla yogurt

½ cup spinach

4 baby carrots

¼ cup protein powder

1 teaspoon flaxseed oil

4 ice cubes

1 tablespoon dry oatmeal

Banana/ Berry Bash

(Serves 2)

6 ice cubes

½ cup apple, orange or juice of your choice

1 ½ bananas

1 ½ cup strawberries

1 sliced orange

1 cup low fat plain or vanilla yogurt

Chapter 7:
Berry Smoothies

For another big boost of antioxidants, without adding a whole lot of unnecessary carbs, add in a half a cup of the berries of your choice. If possible, grow your own berries – I grow my own strawberries and raspberries and they taste a whole lot better than those that you can get commercially. Unfortunately, because they taste so great, they seldom make it to the back door, let alone into my smoothies.

If growing your own is not an option, try to find a local farmer, preferably one that employs organic farming methods and order the berries in bulk – I do this because we eat more berries than what we can produce overall. Buying in bulk is a little bit of work initially – you need to repack and freeze the berries yourself but it usually works out a lot less expensive overall and you have more control over how fresh the berries are.

If neither of the above are an option, or berries are out of season, get yourself some frozen berries so that you always have them on hand. Frozen berries can be mixed in with oatmeal or blended into a smoothie for a real anti-oxidant boost.

Dried berries can be a useful standby if you have no other alternatives. Look for organically produced berries and soak in a basin of water overnight in order to plump them up properly again before you use them.

You do get canned berries but I would really only use these as an absolute last resort as many are canned with sugar, salt and various unhealthy chemicals and additives.

It is also important to switch out the type of berries that you eat from time to time so that you can vary the nutrients contained in your food overall. That means that if you eat blueberries today, try to eat raspberries tomorrow and strawberries the next day, etc.

Berries can also help to regulate blood sugar levels – they are typically lower in sugars and have a high fiber count making them one of the healthiest fruits that you can consume.

The tarter the berries are, the less natural sugar they contain. That said, even sweet berries are lower in natural sugar and so can be enjoyed.

I love a berry smoothie in summer and they are so easy to make.

Nothing as Nice as a Berry Smoothie

(Serves 2)

½ cup strawberries

¾ cup blueberries

½ avocado

2 teaspoon ground flaxseed

1 cup ice cubes

Peach and Blueberry Smoothie

(Serves 2)

1 cup low fat milk or almond milk or soy milk

2 cups sliced peaches (fresh is best, if you cannot get fresh, frozen is okay, failing that, canned is okay as long as it has not been canned in syrup or with added sugar)

1 cup blueberries

Wake Me Up Before You Go Go

(Serves 2)

2 tablespoons Goji berries

2 cups raspberries

2 cups blueberries

3 tablespoons flaxseed powder (or ground flaxseed)

6 ounces plain or vanilla yogurt (low fat)

2 cups purified water or coconut water

No More Wrinkles and Crinkles Smoothie

(Serves 2)

2 cup blueberries

2 medium avocados (peeled and pitted)

2 tablespoons flaxseed (ground if possible)

2 ½ cups coconut water

2 tablespoon honey (or your choice of sweetener)

Minty Berry and Apple Smoothie

(Serves 2)

½ cup mixed berries (frozen or fresh)

10 leaves of mint, freshly picked

1 apple (peeled, sliced and seeds removed)

5 Romaine lettuce leaves, well-rinsed

20 ounces purified water (use juice or coconut water if desired)

Urinary Infection Fighter

(Serves 2)

2 cups purified water or cranberry juice

¾ cup cranberries

1 cucumber (peeled)

1 celery stalk (sliced)

1 ½ apples (peeled, cored and seeds removed)

1 ½ pears (cored)

½ cup spinach

Total Detox

(Serves 2)

2/3 cup frozen cherries (pitted)

1 cup frozen raspberries

1 cup rice milk or almond milk

2 ½ tablespoon honey

1 ½ tablespoon ginger (finely grated)

2 teaspoons flaxseeds

1 tablespoon lemon juice

Chase Away the Blues Smoothie

(Serves 2)

1 ½ cup blueberries

1 ½ cups coconut milk

¾ cup blackberries

¾ cup raspberries

¼ cup Goji berries (These should soak for 10-15 minutes before blending)

2 tablespoon flaxseed (ground)

5 dates (pitted)

2 cups purified water

Oh my Goji Smoothie

(Serves 2)

1 banana

½ cup strawberries (frozen or fresh)

½ cup Goji berries

2 ½ cups coconut water

4 ice cubes

Nourishing, Detox from the Sea

(Serves 2)

1 banana

½ avocado

1 cup almond milk or soymilk

1 cup blueberries

1 tablespoon spirulina powder

½ cup protein powder

2 cups water

Bursting with Berries Smoothie

(Serves 2)

1 cup almond or soy milk

½ cup blackberries

½ cup blueberries

1 banana (frozen)

1 tablespoon honey

1 ½ tablespoon flaxseed

½ cup ice cubes

Carrot and Berry Smoothie

(Serves 2)

1 cup frozen berries (your choice or mixed)

1 cup low fat milk or almond milk

2 cup juice or water

1 ½ carrots

2 tablespoon chia seeds

¼ cup protein powder

Pomegranate and Berry Booster

(Serves 2)

2 cups silken tofu

2 cups pomegranate juice

3 cups mixed berries (fresh or frozen)

¼ cup honey or sweetener of your choice

Lemon and Strawberry Smoothie

(Serves 2)

1 cup strawberries (fresh or frozen)

2 cups full fat milk or soymilk

10 raw almonds

¼ cup lemon juice

1 teaspoon lemon zest

6 ice cubes

A Peach of a Berry Smoothie

(Serves 2)

1 ½ bananas

1 ½ cup strawberries (frozen or fresh)

2 cups low fat milk or soymilk

¼ cup chia seeds

2 tablespoon honey (or your choice of sweetener)

Watermelon Berry Cooler

(Serves 2)

½ cup low fat milk or soymilk

Medium-sized seedless watermelon (scooped out in cubes from rind)

1 cup strawberries (frozen or fresh)

1 cup low fat yogurt

¼ cup protein powder

6 ice cubes

Flaxseed Booster Smoothie

(Serves 2)

1 banana

½ orange (sliced)

½ cup berries (your choice)

½ avocado

1 ½ cups kale or romaine lettuce

1 tablespoon flaxseeds (ground)

1 cup spring water

Sneaky Smoothie

(Serves 2)

½ cup spring water

½ cup orange juice

½ cup strawberries

½ cup blueberries

1 cup kale or spinach (chopped)

Healthy Summer Treat Smoothie

(Serves 2)

1 cup of raspberries

1 cup soy milk

½ cup ice cubes

½ banana

Fruit Fiesta Smoothie

(Serves 2)

1 frozen banana

1 ½ cups peach slices (frozen or fresh)

½ cup blueberries (or strawberries)

1 cup low fat plain or vanilla yogurt

2 tablespoon whey protein powder

½ cup low fat milk or soymilk

Chapter 8:
Spicy Smoothies

With these smoothie recipes, you may be trying something that is a little out of the ordinary for you. In fact, adding spice to a smoothie may seem counter-intuitive but it can be really rewarding in terms of health benefits and flavor as well.

Turmeric: This is actually a wonderful spice that is very popular in India. It is great at treating inflammation and the active ingredient, curcumin, has been found to be as effective an analgesic as aspirin. It is a traditional Indian remedy for treating acid indigestion and heartburn. About a tablespoon daily is enough. Take my advice though and don't take it on an empty stomach. Mix it into your smoothie, cook with it or mix it into a half a glass of milk.

Cinnamon: Cinnamon has been shown to be an effective stabilizer of blood sugar and a valuable ally in the fight against insulin resistance and Type II Diabetes. It is this effect that makes it such a valuable weight loss tool. It has been proven to be as effective in some cases as prescribed diabetes medication. Adding a teaspoon of cinnamon a day is all that is needed to see benefits.

Cayenne Pepper or Chili Pepper: Cayenne Pepper has been proven to stimulate the metabolism, help clear away plaque in the arteries and to help reduce levels of LDL cholesterol (the one you don't want). By stimulating your metabolism, it helps you to lose more weight. In fact, all members of the chili family will help to rev up metabolism and speed up weight loss.

Ginger: Ginger is known to soothe an upset stomach but can also be instrumental when it comes to weight loss – it boosts your metabolism and can work to suppress your appetite as well.

Cardamom: Cardamom is not really a spice that one sees used much outside of curries but this is a pity as it is believed that it can boost the burning of fat within your body.

Fennel: Okay, so fennel is an herb not a spice but I have included it in this section because it has a wonderful soothing effect on the digestive system, helping to ease indigestion and relieve bloating and flatulence.

Ginger Gold

(Serves 2)

½ carrot (sliced)

½ papaya (sliced)

1 orange (sliced)

½ cup pear juice or coconut water

1 teaspoon sliced ginger

½ cup ice cubes

Prune and Cinnamon Smoothie

(Serves 2)

This does have a lot of prunes and fiber in it and so is ideal for when you are feeling constipated.

5 pitted prunes 1 cup ice cubes

1 cup plain yogurt

½ teaspoon cinnamon powder 1 cup apple juice

2 tablespoon honey (if desired for sweetness)

Ginger Antioxidant Kick

(Serves 2)

½ cup blueberries

2 bananas (fresh or frozen)

4 ice cubes

½ cup ginger juice

2 ½ cups soy milk (almond milk or low calorie milk is fine)

Cucumber Cilantro Cooler

(Serves 2)

½ cucumber (sliced)

1 cup kale (or romaine lettuce or spinach)

1 ½ cups spring water

1/3 cup cilantro (chopped)

½ lemon (peeled and de-seeded)

1 wedge lime (peeled and de-seeded)

½ cup cilantro

Jicama Smoothie

(Serves 2)

1 lime

1 cucumber

1 apple

10 Romaine leaves

1 avocado

1 cup jicama (grated or sliced)

½ cup cilantro

½ cup protein powder

3 pitted dates

2 ½ cups water

Carrot and Tomato Booster Smoother

(Serves 2)

2-3 tomatoes

5 carrots

2 bell peppers (preferably red – sliced and seeds removed)

3 garlic cloves

3 celery stalks

1 cup spinach

1 red jalapeno (seeds removed)

½ cup water cress

Flu Fighting Smoothie

(Serves 2)

1 carrot

½ beet (chopped)

1 celery stalk (chopped)

½ cucumber (peeled and sliced)

1 tablespoon of sliced ginger

1 teaspoon minced garlic

1 cup ice cubes, ½ cup spring water

Evergreen Smoothie

(Serves 2)

1 cup kale or spinach (chopped)

1 apple (peeled, sliced, deseeded)

½ cup seedless grapes (green)

1 kiwi (sliced and peeled)

1 cup honeydew melon (shopped and peeled)

½ teaspoon of Cayenne Pepper

As Good as Apple Pie

(Serves 2)

¼ cup caramel sauce

1 cup low fat vanilla yogurt 2 cups apple juice

1 tablespoon cinnamon

2 tablespoon sweetener (your choice)

6 ice cubes

Banana Cream

(Serves 2)

1 cup low fat vanilla yogurt

1 ½ bananas

2 cups vanilla almond milk

½ cup low fat cottage cheese

¼ cup cream cheese (low fat is okay)

½ teaspoon cinnamon

Banana and Pumpkin Booster

1 ½ cup soymilk or low fat milk

6 kale leaves

2 tablespoon flaxseed oil

1 ½ banana

½ teaspoon cinnamon

1 cup pumpkin puree (canned is fine)

6 ice cubes

Veggie and Spice and All Things Nice

1 cup avocado

¼ cup lemon juice

14 ounces carrot juice

Dash of cayenne pepper

1 ½ tablespoon fresh ginger (grated)

6 ice cubes

Raspberry Treat

(Serves 2)

10 ounces plain or vanilla low fat yogurt

1 cup low fat, skim milk or soymilk

½ cup dark chocolate chips

1 ½ cups raspberries (frozen or fresh)

1 ½ cup raspberry juice

6 ice cubes

A dash of chili powder (optional but makes for a really great flavor sensation)

Kale and Ginger Stunner

(Serves 2)

1 cup kale or spinach or romaine lettuce

1 apple (peeled, sliced and de-seeded)

¼ bunch parsley

½ cucumber (peeled and sliced)

1 celery stalk (chopped)

½ lemon (peeled, sliced and de-seeded)

2 teaspoon ginger (chopped)

1 cup spring water

Bloody Mary Smoothie

½ cup apple juice

1 cup tomato juice

1 ½ cups chopped tomatoes

2/3 cup chopped carrots

2/3 cup chopped celery

2/3 teaspoon hot sauce

9 ice cubes

Blueberry Smoothie

(Serves 2)

2/3 cup soy protein

1 large banana

½ cup frozen blueberries 1 tablespoon flaxseed oil

16 ounces water

1 tablespoon honey or sweetener of your choice

1 teaspoon cinnamon

6 ice cubes (if desired)

Something Yummy is Coming

1 ½ cups frozen mixed berries

½ banana

6 ice cubes

1 ½ cups plain or vanilla low fat yogurt (or milk, low fat)

1 tablespoon sweetener (your choice)

1 tablespoon turmeric

Awesome Peanut Butter Smoothie

1 banana

1 ¼ cup low fat milk (or soy milk)

2/3 cup smooth peanut butter (low fat preferably)

2 tablespoon protein powder

1 teaspoon cinnamon powder

8 ice cubes

Apple Dessert Smoothie

(Serves 2)

12 ounces plain or vanilla low fat yogurt

1 cup of low fat milk or soymilk

2 teaspoon apple pie spice

2 sliced apples (use your favorite kind)

4 tablespoon almond or cashew butter

8 ice cubes

Pineapple and Fennel Stomach Soother

(Serves 2)

½ ounce fresh mint (chopped)

½ avocado (sliced)

½ cup fennel (chopped)

½ cup pineapple (crushed from can is ok or fresh sliced) 1 cup spring water

½ cup ice cubes

Chapter 9:
Smoothies for Weight Loss

Get Ready for Weight Loss

1 ½ bananas

1 ½ cup spinach (chopped)

¼ cup avocado (peeled and pit removed)

2 tablespoon sunflower seeds

¼ cup lemon juice (no seeds)

2 ½ cups soy or almond milk (low fat dairy milk is okay too)

3 tablespoon sweetener (your choice)

Green Tea and Strawberry Smoothie

(Serves 2)

2 tablespoons green tea powder

1 ½ bananas, 3 cups strawberries

2 cups coconut water

3 tablespoon chia seeds

¼ cup plain yogurt

2 tablespoon sweetener (honey or your choice).

Cleanse From the Inside Out

This one will get your system working and in a relatively short amount of time.

The Epsom salts pull water into the colon, which in turn makes it much easier to go to the restroom.

After this smoothie you should sort of hang around the house for a while!

½ cup applesauce

½ cup plain yogurt

1 tablespoon Epsom salt

½ cup spring water

½ banana

½ cup ice cubes

5 pitted prunes

Hard to Beet

(Serves 2)

1 medium sized beet (cleaned and sliced)

2 apples (peeled, sliced and seeds and core removed)

1/3 cup parsley

2 tablespoon chia seeds

¾ inch of ginger

1 ½ lemons (peeled, sliced and seeds removed)

2 cups kale leaves (chopped)

16 ounces purified water

Cilantro Detox Smoothie

(Serves 2)

½ avocado (sliced)

¼ lemon (peeled and de-seeded)

½ pear

¼ cucumber (peeled and sliced)

1 cup kale (or romaine lettuce)

½ ounces sliced ginger

2 ounces protein powder (hemp or pea)

3 tablespoon cilantro (chopped)

Kale and Mango System Cleanser

(Serves 2)

1 ½ cups orange juice

¼ cup chopped parsley

1 ½ chopped celery stems 1 ½ cups cubed mango

1 ½ cups chopped kale leaves

To Lose Water Weight Fast

(Serves 2)

1 cup kale (or romaine lettuce)

1 cup orange juice

½ cup mango (sliced)

¼ cup parsley (chopped)

1 stalk celery (chopped)

Zesty Apple Smoothie

1 ½ lemons (peeled, sliced and seeds removed)

2 apples (green preferably)

1 cucumber (peeled)

5 leaves of red lettuce

½ cup mango cubes (frozen or fresh)

2 teaspoon barley grass powder

16 ounces purified water

Kale and Apple Energy Booster

2 cups kale or spinach

½ cup Greek yogurt

½ cup apple or orange juice (unsweetened and de-seeded)

5 teaspoon flaxseeds

2 teaspoon maple syrup 1 cup ice cubes

Lime Soul Soother

½ cup lime juice

1 cup almond milk 1 banana (frozen)

1 ½ cups kale (or spinach)

5 ice cubes

2 tablespoon almond butter (or sunflower butter)

2 pitted dates

Avocado Smoothie from Heaven

½ avocado

½ banana

2 tablespoon honey

1 cup ice cubes

½ cup spring water 1/3 cup lime juice 1 tablespoon chai seeds

½ mango (peeled, pitted and cubed)

Quick Weight Loss Smoothie

(Serves 2)

1 Granny Smith apple (sliced and de-seeded)

½ pear

1 celery stalk (chopped)

1 cup kale

1 tablespoon ginger

1 cup ice cubes

½ cup spring water or apple juice

Be a Mean Fat-Burning Machine

(Serves 2)

1 cup of kale or spinach (chopped)

1 stalk of celery (chopped)

1 apple (sliced)

1 tablespoon lemon juice

1/3 cucumber (sliced)

1 cup ice cubes

¼ cup spring water

Banana Shake with a Wake up Factor

(Serves 2)

1 ½ bananas

2 cups coffee (cold)

½ cup protein powder

½ cup low fat milk or soymilk

½ cup dry oats

Peach and Chia Smoothie

(Serves 2)

1 ½ cups sliced frozen or fresh peaches

1 tablespoon chia seeds soaked overnight in enough water to cover them

1 ½ cups low fat or non-fat milk 4 ice cubes

3 tablespoons sweetener (of your choice)

Kick into Gear Smoothie

(Serves 2)

4 teaspoons cocoa powder 2 shots espresso

1 cup low-fat plain or vanilla yogurt

2 tablespoons chia seeds

2 tablespoons sweetener (of your choice)

6 ice cubes

Mango Bliss

(Serves 2)

1 cup mango juice (bottled is fine)

2 tablespoon sweetener (of your choice)

2 tablespoons lime or lemon juice (preferably freshly squeezed

5 ice cubes

½ cup mashed ripe avocado

½ cup plain or vanilla low fat yogurt

½ cup mangoes – cubed

On Your Way to the Tropics Smoothie

8 ounces pineapple chunks (canned is fine if you cannot find fresh, as long as you choose the unsweetened variety and also add the juice to the smoothie)

1 cup low fat milk or soymilk

½ cup coconut water

½ cup fresh coconut flesh

2 tablespoons flaxseed oil

8 ice cubes

3 tablespoons sweetener (of your choice)

Get Up and Go Recipe

(Serves 2)

1 ½ oranges (peeled and sectioned)

3 tablespoon honey (or your choice of sweetener)

8 ice cubes

1 cup low fat milk or soymilk

Nutty as a Banana Smoothie

(Serves 2)

1 tablespoon cashew butter

1 ½ banana

1 tablespoon flaxseed oil

1 cup low fat yogurt (plain or vanilla)

3 tablespoon sweetener (of your choice)

1 tablespoon vanilla extract

The Joy of Citrus Smoothie

(Serves 2)

12 ounces citrus flavored yogurt (of your choice)

2 oranges peeled and cut into pieces

1½ cups soymilk or low fat milk

1½ tablespoon flaxseed oil

8 ice cubes

Chapter 10:

Your Smoothie Cheat Sheet to Keep Your Kitchen Stocked

The great thing about smoothies is that you can easily whip them up from your everyday foods – foods that you probably already keep in the house anyway. That said, there are one or two other things that you may consider adding so let's go through the list and see where we stand, shall we?

Liquids

Your smoothie is going to need some form of liquid to make it easier to drink. You can pretty much choose anything from water to juice. I am also going to include ice here because it will, eventually, melt.

Water: I drink about 12 to 14 glasses of water a day anyway, so when it comes to my smoothies, I prefer to add a liquid that has a bit more substance or flavor. Generally speaking, if I do add fruit juice, I will usually dilute it with water to reduce the overall sugar content of the smoothie.

Coconut Water: Coconut water has a range of electrolytes and nutrients in it and it does not have an overwhelming flavor. It is great for smoothies where you already have an alternative protein source in the ingredients.

Milk: You will see that I do use a lot of milk in my smoothies but that I do not just limit myself to one type of milk – I do use dairy milk, almond milk and other non-dairy alternatives such as soy. Personally, I love the creamy goodness of dairy milk but do find that I have to be careful not drink too much of it or I get a runny nose. I do also love almond milk because it tastes great and is so easy to make. What I like about having milk in my smoothies is that it ups the protein content, helping me to feel fuller for longer.

Fruit Juice: You will have noticed that there are not many smoothie recipes in this book that feature fruit juices. Fruit juices should be reserved as an occasional treat because they can contain as much sugar as soda. If you decide that you would rather have fruit juices than milk, please dilute the fruit juice with an equal quantity of water.

Herbal Teas: Herbal teas are a better option to fruit juice and can also be very beneficial as a base to your smoothie. Peppermint tea, for example, will make a great after-dinner smoothie or a breakfast smoothie for someone who needs to focus throughout the day. Chamomile tea can be used as a base for a soothing smoothie for someone who is over-anxious.

Green Tea as a Base

Green tea is the best health drink that there is and deserves special mention. It is high in anti-oxidants and other nutrients and will help to, amongst other things, increase the amount of fat lost, reduce your risk of developing cancer and increase the level at which your brain functions as well.

There are a host of benefits – we do nowhere near fully understand everything that green tea can do. But here I will list the benefits that have been scientifically proven:

A lot of the bioactive compounds survive the process from tea leave to teacup. The most important of these are the antioxidants. Antioxidants help to prevent free radicals forming. Fewer free radicals mean less damage to your system. You will not appear to age as fast and will be less likely to pick up diseases.

Cancer is still one of the biggest killers of our age. It has now been established that damage caused by oxidation is a big contributor when it comes to the growth of cancerous cells. Oxidation is caused by free radicals and these can be neutralized by antioxidants. For maximum protection, skip the milk – milk lowers the number of antioxidants present.

Adult onset diabetes has now been rated a global epidemic and affects hundreds of millions of people. The disease is characterized by high levels of blood sugar and the inability of the body to cope because insulin effectiveness is reduced.

Green tea has been shown to help improve the body's sensitivity to insulin and to lower the levels of sugar in the blood. A study in Japan found that you could decrease you chances of developing Adult Onset Diabetes by as much as 42%. Studies show that green tea can improve insulin sensitivity and reduce blood sugar

Cardiovascular diseases are the biggest mass murderers the world has seen. Green tea reduces your risk of being a victim by improving your statistics where it matters – your LDL cholesterol, overall cholesterol and triglyceride levels. Because of the antioxidant abilities of green tea, LDL cholesterol is less likely to become oxidized. This is a big one when it comes to cardiovascular disease. Drinking green tea regularly, without milk, reduces your chances of cardiovascular disease by as much as 31%.

Catechins have anti-bacterial and anti-viral actions as well. This is good news for you teeth – the tea can decrease the growth rate of the plaque-forming bacteria in the mouth. It also helps fight bad breath.

Fruits

As far as fruits go, you can choose whichever fruits you prefer. I do suggest using fruits that are in season as far as possible, the fresher the better. The advantage of having your fruit in smoothie format as opposed to juicing format is that you get all the fiber as well.

Apples: Vitamin A, C, D, iron, Calcium and magnesium.

Bananas: One of the most common ingredients in the smoothie world. Use to give a great creamy texture and sweet flavor to your smoothie.

Blueberries – Flavorful and chock-full of antioxidants.

Dates: Sweet and full of amino acids and fiber. Pears – Antioxidant.

Goji berries: Aids in well-being, quality of sleep and weight control.

Kiwi: Loaded with Vitamin C.

Mangos: Vitamin C, A, B6, GABA and lots of fiber.

Papaya: Vitamin C, D, B6 and A, along with iron, magnesium and calcium.

Pineapple: Vitamin C, A and B complex, along with manganese and copper.

Raspberries: Antioxidant and anti-inflammatory.

Strawberries: Vitamin C and plenty of minerals. Oranges – Vitamin C and fiber.

Greens

These greens are considered Superfoods, along with many of the fruits listed above. Superfoods are simply 'Exceptional" foods that have exceptional nutritional properties, which are thought to be highly beneficial for our health.

Kale: Has Vitamin C and A, and some important flavonoids.

Spinach: Vitamin K, C, Beta-carotene, iron, magnesium, calcium and protein.

Swiss chard: Vitamin E and C and is an antioxidant. Dandelion greens – Vitamin C, B6, potassium, calcium and iron. Cilantro – Tasty and is a detoxifier.

Bok Choy: Vitamin A, C, K, magnesium, potassium, manganese, calcium and iron.

Mint leaves: Refreshing and antioxidant, giving energy and soothing digestive upsets.

A Note on Fiber

Fruits and vegetables provide fiber. Fiber is essential if you want to lose weight and maintain the weight loss. If you are not getting enough fiber, you can have as much as 4-8lbs of undigested food sluggishly moving around in your intestines.

There are beneficial bacteria in the colon that help us to digest the food and get all the goodness we can from it.

Without enough fiber, the "bad" bacteria soon overrun these good little soldiers.

Instead of the nutrients being taken out of the food, it literally rots in your gut. This causes gas to develop and you start bloating.

Your body does not get the nutrients it needs so you are hungrier and eat more and the whole cycle starts again.

The rotting food is not only causing you troubles with your weight though – toxins released by the fermentation process are being absorbed into your blood stream and putting you at risk for serious health issues.

There are two types of fiber – soluble and insoluble. We need both.

The body can digest soluble fiber and it helps to mop up the dangerous LDL cholesterol in your blood and helps to keep blood sugar levels in check.

The body does not absorb insoluble fiber but it helps keep the food moving at a steady pace through the digestive tract.

It also helps you feel fuller faster.

Think about it for a second. How many oranges can you eat in one sitting – imagine that they are your favorite food – before you feel full?

Now take the fiber away – like they do when they make orange juice.

Did you know that to get one cup of pure orange juice, you need to squeeze 22 oranges?

That is not cost effective for the makers of the juice though so they dilute it with denatured juice and add sugar so it tastes better.

Your cup of orange juice is about the equivalent of eating 6 oranges with almost the same amount of sugar as you will find in a glass of coke.

Take the fiber out and it is easy to get your 5 – 9 portions of fruit and vegetables a day.

The problem is that without the fiber, there is nothing to slow down the body's absorption of the sugar and your sugar levels spike.

Your body also doesn't register the calories because they are liquid so it won't help you feel fuller either.

The net result is that you may as well be drinking sugar – what's left of the vitamins in that juice will never outweigh the dangerous sugar rush.

Nuts Seeds and Other Essentials

All you need is 75g of nuts a day to see the benefits. Eat them over and above your normal protein intake and you'll get a healthy boost. They are calorie dense but it should be remembered that they contain loads of nutrients and monounsaturated fats. Nuts will also help you feel full, give you an energy boost and keep your blood levels more stable.

Almonds: full of protein and fiber and great for boosting energy and satiating hunger. **Cashews**: Low fat and high in minerals.

Walnuts: Vitamin E, flavonoids and is good for the heart.

Chia seeds: Low calorie, high in fiber, protein and minerals.

Flaxseeds: Antioxidant and high in fiber.

Pumpkin seeds: High in Omega-3 fatty acids and a range of nutrients

Protein Powder

Protein powders have long been used by people on low carb diets in order to help fuel their bodies and build muscle. Protein powder – usually in the form of whey powder or soy powder is a great ingredient to add to your shakes. It will give you more energy, help you to feel full for longer and will also help you to burn more calories.

Sweeteners

I have included a lot of recipes that allow you to add a sweetener of your choice. Personally, when making my smoothies, I ensure that I use enough fruit so that it is sweet enough and try to avoid sweeteners. That said, there are times when a bit of sweetness is necessary.

I advise using either honey or stevia to sweeten your smoothies if you feel that you need to. Xylitol is okay as a second choice.

In terms or real sugar, black strap molasses can be used but do completely avoid refined sugar and artificial sweeteners.

Conclusion

Thank you again for downloading this book!

I truly hope that this book has shown you how to make your own superfood smoothies and given you the knowledge that you need to come up with your own exciting variants.

Please consider this book as an introduction into this exciting world and use it as a basis to build your skills in future. I encourage you to read more on superfoods and to learn more about them as you go along. If you enjoyed this book, look out for other titles in my Superfoods for Healthy Living series available on Amazon.

All that is left now is to practice what you have learned in this book and apply it to your daily life! Smoothie anyone?

Finally, I would really appreciate it if you could take the time to review this book on Amazon for me. I would love to read your thoughts and it will help me to continue helping others to become healthy and happy.

Thank you and good luck!

www.ingramcontent.com/pod-product-compliance
Lightning Source LLC
Chambersburg PA
CBHW072204280526
45788CB00002B/873